Resistance
Band Workouts
For
Beginners

A Quick and Convenient Exercise to Getting Fit and Developing Strength While at Home and on the Go.

Robert H. McCarthy

All rights reserved. No part of this book may be reproduced or used in any manner without the written permission of the copyright owner except for the use of quotation in a book review. Copyright © **Robert H. McCarthy** 2023

Table of contents

INTRODUCTION   **5**

What are resistance bands?   9

Benefits of using resistance bands   9

Chapter 1: Getting Started with Resistance Band Workouts   **12**

Choosing the Right Resistance Bands   13

How to Use Resistance Bands Safely   14

Creating a Resistance Band Workout Routine   15

Chapter 2: Upper Body Exercises   **17**

Shoulder Exercises   17

Arm Exercises   21

Back Exercises   23

Chapter 3: Lower Body Exercises   **25**

Quadriceps Exercises   25

Hamstring Exercises   29

Glute Exercises   31

Chapter 4: Core Exercises   **35**

Plank Exercises   35

Crunch Exercises   37

Chapter 5: Workout Routines   **41**

Beginner Workout Routine   41

Intermediate Workout Routine   42

Advanced Workout Routine   43

Chapter 6: Tips and Troubleshooting   **46**

    Tips for Enhancing Resistance Band Workouts   46

    Troubleshooting Common Challenges   48

Conclusion   **50**

    Embracing Consistency and Achieving Fitness
    Goals   50

    The Importance of Consistency   50

    Tracking Your Progress   51

    Setting Realistic Goals   51

Fitness journal   **53**

INTRODUCTION

Amidst the chaos and clutter of a bustling flea market, amidst the throngs of eager bargain hunters and the cacophony of voices, a weathered book lay forgotten, its pages yellowed with age and its cover bearing the scars of countless journeys. It was a book titled "Resistance Band Workouts for Beginners," its significance lost amidst the sea of trinkets and treasures.

One fateful afternoon, a young woman named Sarah stumbled upon the inconspicuous book. Intrigued by its title, she picked it up, her fingers brushing against the worn cover. Sarah, a creature of habit, had grown increasingly frustrated with her sedentary lifestyle and the lackluster results of her occasional gym visits.

She yearned for a change, a spark that would ignite her fitness journey.

As Sarah delved into the pages of the book, she discovered a treasure trove of knowledge and guidance. The book outlined the benefits of resistance band workouts, their versatility, and their effectiveness for individuals of all fitness levels. Sarah was captivated by the simplicity and accessibility of the exercises, realizing that she could transform her living room into a personal gym.

With newfound enthusiasm, Sarah set out to implement the principles of the book. She purchased a set of resistance bands, eager to experience the transformative power of these versatile tools. Guided by the clear instructions and illustrations, Sarah began her journey, her living room becoming her sanctuary of self-improvement.

The first few workouts were challenging, as Sarah's muscles protested against the unaccustomed strain. Yet, she persevered, her determination fueled by the promise of a healthier and stronger body. She embraced the discomfort, viewing it as a sign of progress, a testament to her unwavering commitment.

As the days turned into weeks, Sarah noticed subtle changes in her body. Her muscles began to tone and define, her posture improved, and she felt more energized throughout the day. The book had become her companion, a source of inspiration and guidance.

The physical changes were not the only transformations Sarah experienced. Resistance band workouts became a cathartic outlet, a release valve for the stresses and anxieties of daily life. As she focused on each exercise, her mind became clear, her thoughts unburdened by the worries of the world.

Sarah's newfound dedication to her physical well-being spilled over into other aspects of her life. She adopted healthier eating habits, prioritizing nutritious foods that fueled her body and mind. She embraced a more mindful approach to her daily activities, seeking balance and harmony in all aspects of her life.

The book had become more than just a guide to resistance band workouts; it had become a catalyst for personal transformation. Sarah had discovered the profound connection between physical fitness and overall well-being, realizing that true strength lies not just in the muscles but also in the mind and spirit.

What are resistance bands?

Resistance bands, commonly known as fitness bands or workout bands, are elastic bands that create varying resistance against your motions. Unlike conventional free weights, which depend on gravity for force, resistance bands provide a more constant and regulated kind of resistance across the whole range of motion. This unique trait makes resistance bands a perfect option for persons of all fitness levels, from beginners to seasoned athletes.

Benefits of using resistance bands

Resistance bands are a terrific method to add strength training to your exercise program. They provide a variety of advantages over conventional weights, including:

Versatility: Resistance bands may be used to do a broad range of workouts, from upper body and lower body to core and cardio.

Portability: Resistance bands are lightweight and simple to pack, making them suitable for home workouts, vacation, or outdoor activities.

Affordability: Resistance bands are fairly economical compared to typical weightlifting equipment.

Safety: Resistance bands are less prone to cause accidents than conventional weights since they offer a more continuous and regulated resistance.

Functional training: Resistance bands may be used to produce functional motions that replicate daily tasks, such as squatting, lunging, and rowing.

Muscle activation: Resistance bands may aid to activate more muscle fibers than conventional weights since they offer resistance throughout the whole range of motion of an activity.

Improved flexibility: Resistance bands may assist to enhance flexibility since they offer a mild stretch to the muscles.

Rehabilitation: Resistance bands are widely used in physical therapy to help patients recover from injuries.

suitable for all ages and fitness levels: Resistance bands are suitable for individuals of all ages and fitness levels, since you may adjust the resistance to your own requirements.

Chapter 1: Getting Started with Resistance Band Workouts

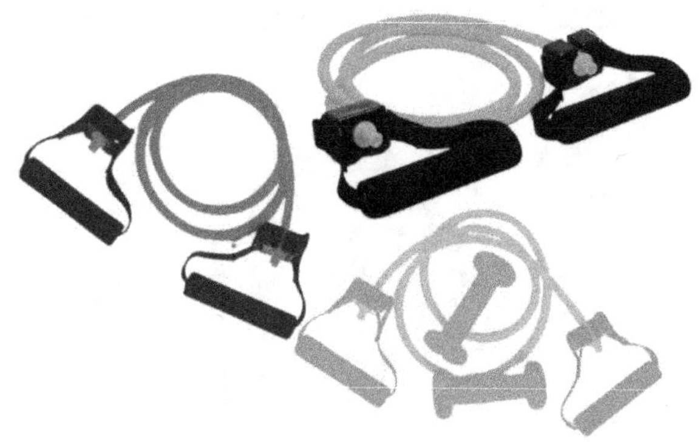

Choosing the Right Resistance Bands

With a variety of resistance bands available, picking the optimum amount of resistance is vital for a good exercise. Resistance bands are often color-coded to show their resistance degree, ranging from low to heavy.

Beginners: For individuals new to resistance band exercises, beginning with light-resistance bands is suggested. This enables you to progressively increase strength and familiarize yourself with the workouts before moving on to stronger resistance bands.

Intermediate: As your strength develops, you may advance to medium-resistance bands. These bands give a harder challenge, helping you further increase your strength and muscular tone.

Advanced: Experienced users may employ heavy-resistance bands for optimum challenge and muscular activation.

How to Use Resistance Bands Safely

To guarantee a safe and successful exercise, it's crucial to follow appropriate technique while utilizing resistance bands. Here are some essential tips:

Maintain good form: Pay attention to your body alignment and posture during each exercise to minimize strain or injury.

Use a regulated tempo: Avoid jerky or sudden motions. Maintain a calm and controlled speed during each exercise.

Listen to your body: Rest when required and prevent overexertion. If you encounter discomfort, cease the workout immediately.

Inspect the bands regularly: Check the bands for cracks or rips before each usage. Replace any broken bands quickly.

Creating a Resistance Band Workout Routine

Designing a tailored resistance band training plan is vital for accomplishing your fitness objectives. Consider your fitness level, objectives, and available time while developing your regimen.

Frequency: Aim for 2-3 resistance band exercises each week, allowing for enough rest and recuperation between sessions.

Time: Start with shorter exercises and progressively increase the time as your fitness improves.

Exercise Selection: Choose exercises that target all main muscle groups in your body.

Range: Incorporate a range of activities to make your training tough and entertaining.

Progression: Gradually increase the resistance or repetitions as your strength develops.

Resistance bands provide a varied, effective, and handy approach to boost your workout experience. With a large selection of workouts available and the option to modify resistance levels, resistance bands may be personalized to people of different fitness levels and objectives. Embrace the variety of resistance bands and go on a road to attaining your fitness ambitions.

Chapter 2: Upper Body Exercises

This chapter gives a complete overview to upper body workouts utilizing resistance bands. These exercises are meant to target the main muscular groups in the upper body, including the shoulders, arms, and back.

Shoulder Exercises

Shoulder Press

Stand with your feet hip-width apart and grasp a resistance band in each hand at your shoulders. Press the bands up above until your arms are straight. Slowly lower the bands back to your shoulders.

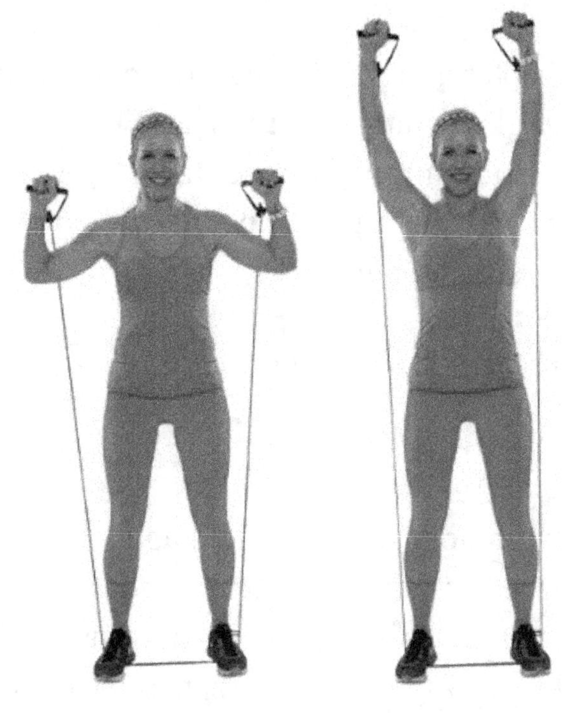

Lateral Raises

Stand with your feet hip-width apart and grip a resistance band in each hand with your hands facing down. Raise the bands out to the sides until your arms are parallel to the floor. Slowly drop the bands back down to your sides.

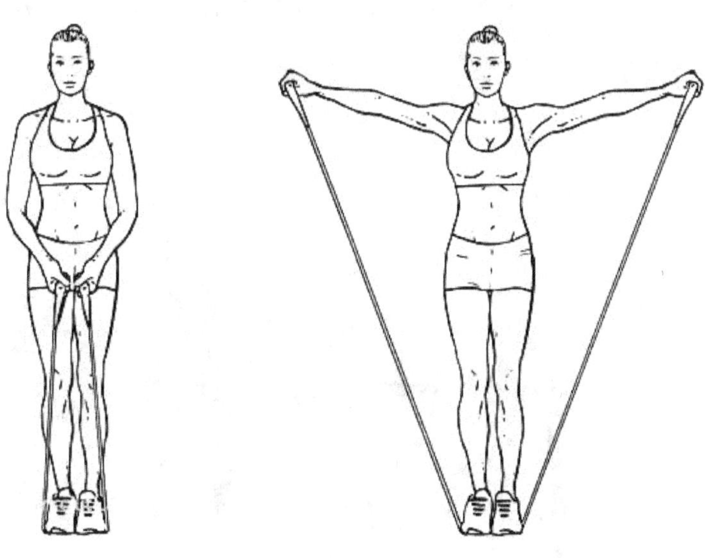

Rear Delt Flyes

Stand with your feet hip-width apart and grip a resistance band behind your head with both hands. Bend your elbows slightly and maintain your back straight. Spread your arms out to the sides until your elbows are level with your shoulders. Slowly lower the bands back to your head.

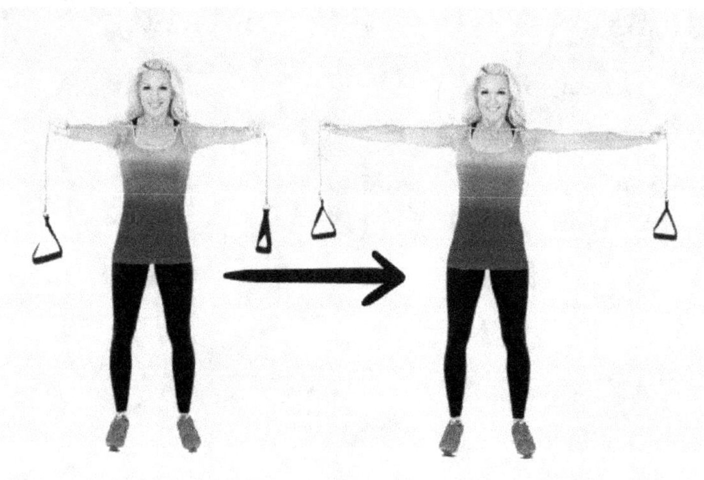

Arm Exercises

Bicep Curls

Stand with your feet hip-width apart and grip a resistance band in each hand with your palms facing up. Curl the bands up towards your shoulders, and then gently drop them back down.

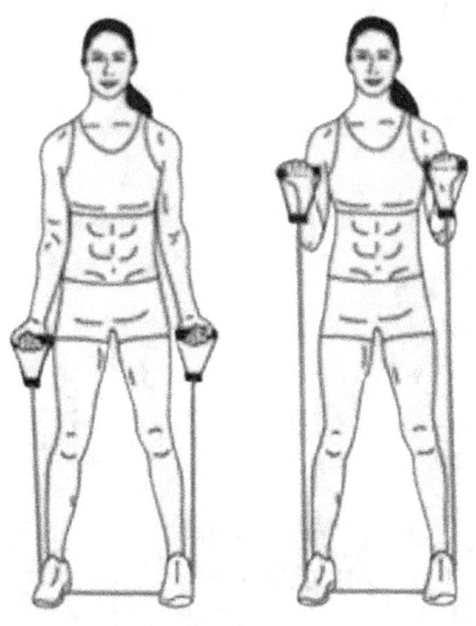

Tricep Extensions

Stand with your feet hip-width apart and grip a resistance band behind your head with both hands. Extend your arms behind you until they are straight. Slowly lower the band back to your head.

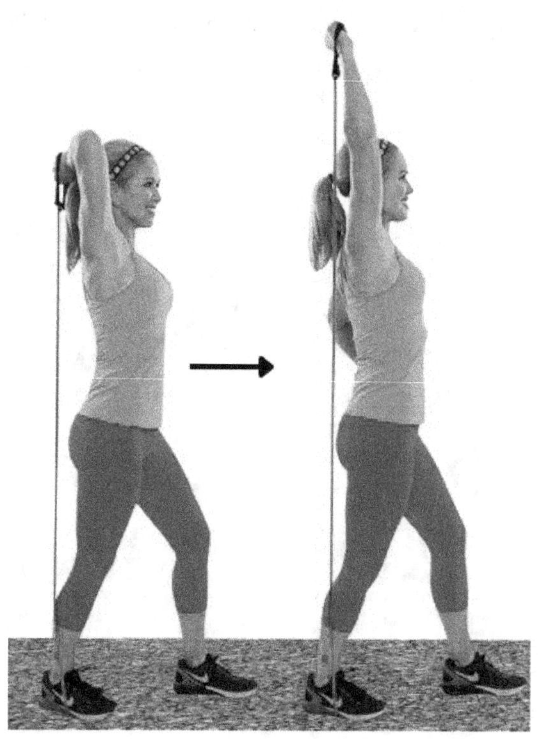

Back Exercises

Bent-Over Rows

Stand with your feet hip-width apart and bend forward at the waist, maintaining your back straight. Hold a resistance band in each hand with your palms facing down. Row the bands up towards your chest, and then gently drop them back down.

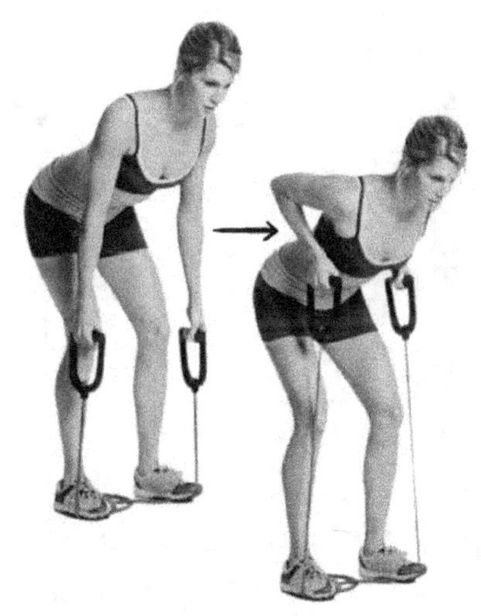

Face Pulls

Stand with your feet hip-width apart and grip a resistance band in each hand with your hands facing down. Bring the bands up towards your face, keeping your elbows close to your head. Slowly drop the bands back down to your sides.

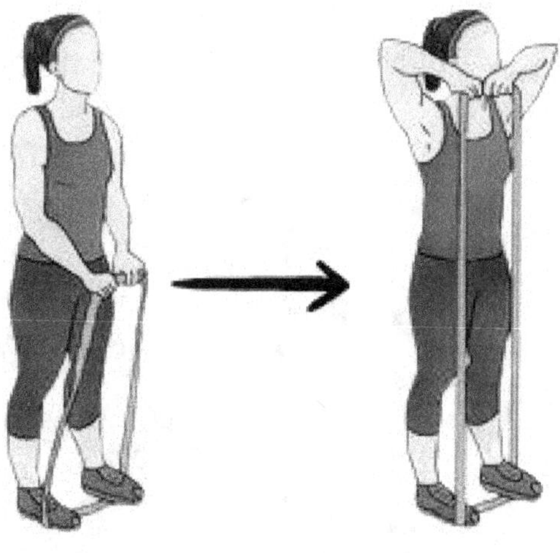

By adding these exercises into your training program, you may efficiently target the main muscle groups in your upper body, boosting your strength, muscular tone, and overall fitness.

Chapter 3: Lower Body Exercises

These exercises are meant to target all main muscular groups in the lower body, including the quadriceps, hamstrings, glutes, and calves.

Quadriceps Exercises

Squats

Stand with your feet hip-width apart and wrap a resistance band around your ankles. Squat down as if you are sitting in a chair, and then gently rise back up.

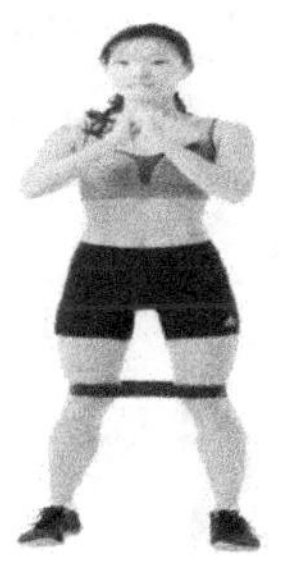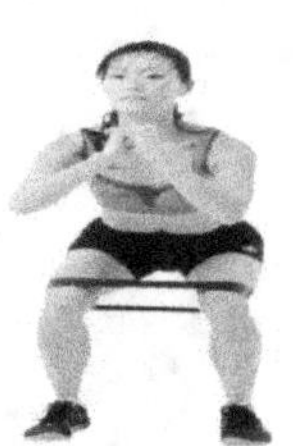

Lunges

Stand with your feet hip-width apart and wrap a resistance band around your leg.

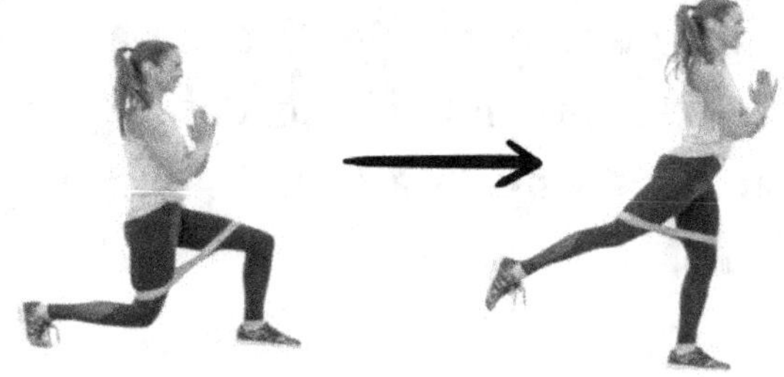

Leg Press

Lie on your back on a bench with your feet flat on the floor and a resistance band around your ankles. Press your heels into the floor to stretch your legs until your knees are straight. Slowly drop your heels back to the floor.

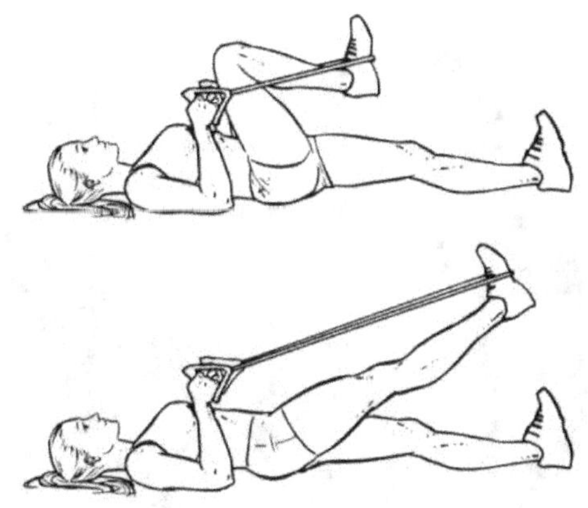

Leg Extensions

Sit on a leg extension machine with a resistance band around your ankles. Extend your legs until they are straight, and then gently drop them back to the starting position.

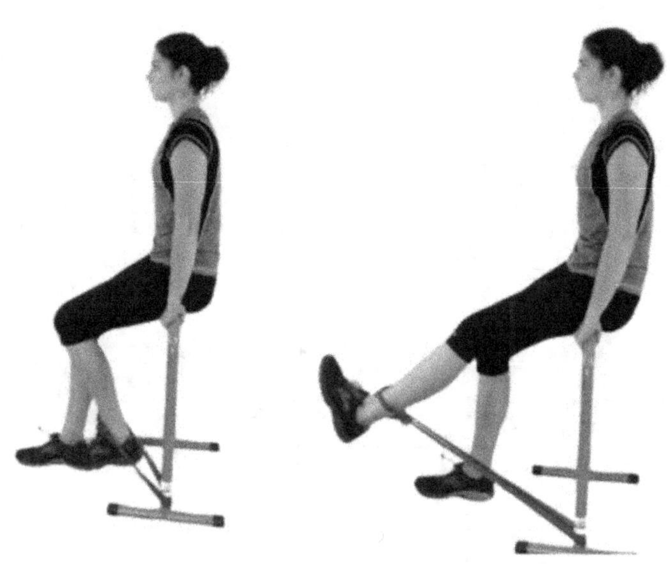

Hamstring Exercises

Deadlifts

Stand with your feet shoulder-width apart and grasp a resistance band in each hand. Keep your back straight and your knees slightly bent. Lower the band towards your feet, and then gently stand back up.

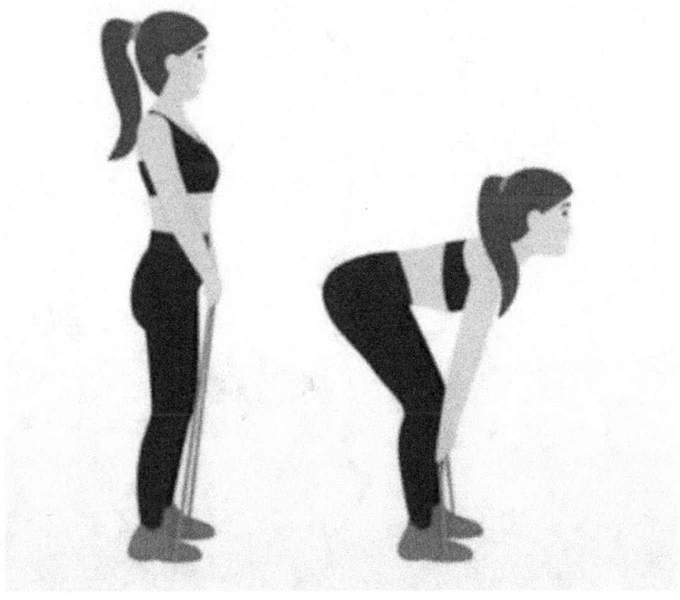

Hamstring Curls

Lie on your back on a bench with a resistance band around your ankles. Bend your knees and bring your heels towards your glutes. Slowly drop your heels back to the floor.

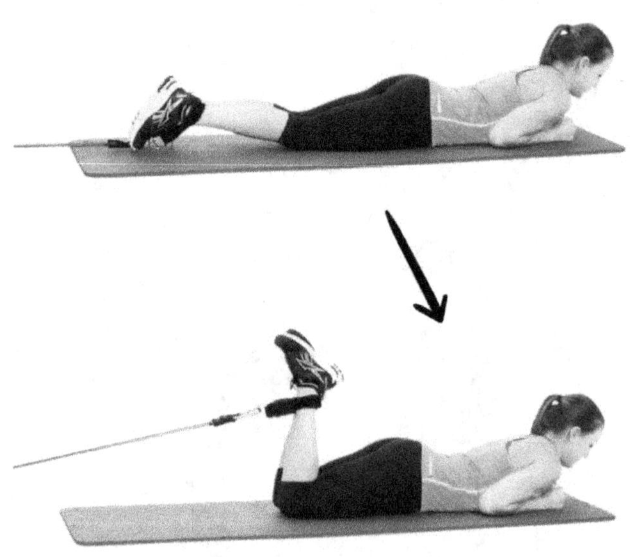

Glute Exercises

Glute Bridges

Lie on your back on the floor with your knees bent and your feet flat on the floor. Loop a resistance band around your ankles. Lift your hips off the floor until your body creates a straight line from your shoulders to your knees. Slowly drop your hips back to the floor.

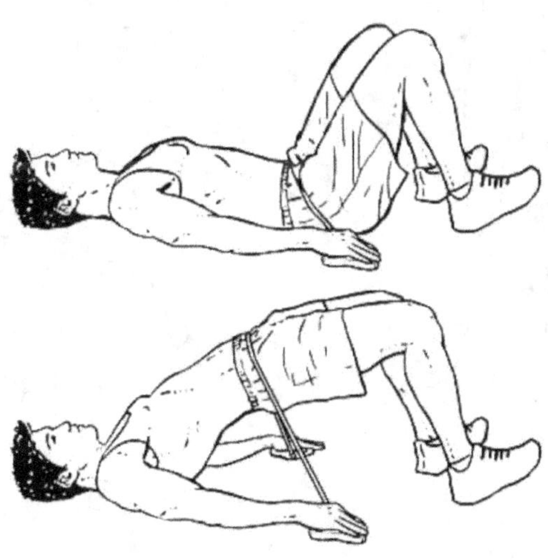

Hip Abduction

Stand with your feet hip-width apart and wrap a resistance band around your ankles. Step out to the side with your right leg, and then gently step back to the starting position. Repeat with your left leg.

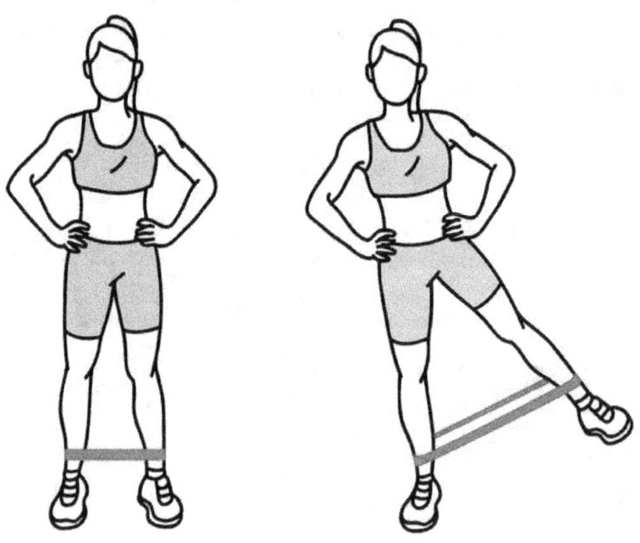

Calf Exercises

Calf Raises Stand with your feet shoulder-width apart and thread a resistance band around the balls of your feet. Stand on your toes, and then gently drop your heels back down to the floor.

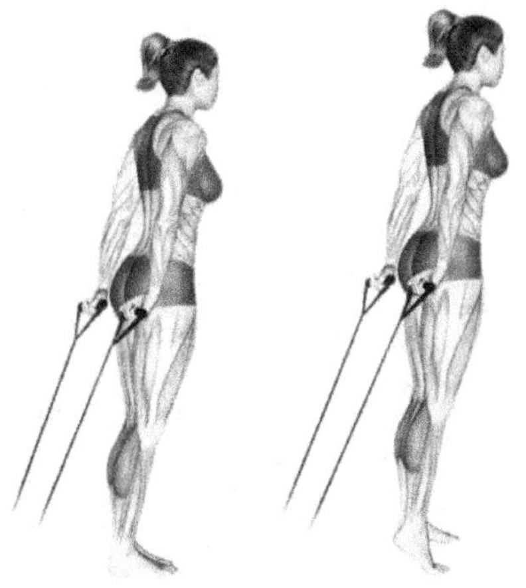

By adding these exercises into your training program, you may efficiently target the main muscle groups in your lower body, boosting your strength, muscular tone, and general fitness.

Chapter 4: Core Exercises

A strong core is vital for general stability, balance, and injury prevention. Resistance bands provide a diverse and efficient technique to target the core muscles, including the rectus abdominis, transverse abdominis, and obliques. This chapter gives a complete overview of core workouts with resistance bands.

Plank Exercises

Plank

Start in a push-up stance with your forearms on the floor and your elbows aligned beneath your shoulders. Keep your body in a straight line from head to toe. Hold the position for as long as possible.

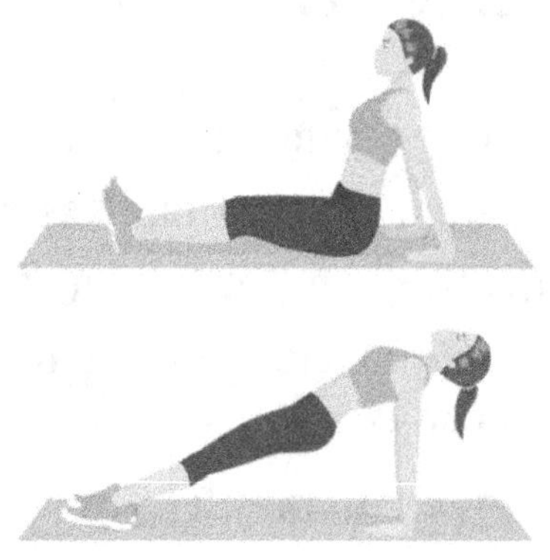

Side Plank

Start in a side plank posture with your forearm on the floor and your elbow aligned beneath your shoulder. Keep your body in a straight line from head to toe, stacking your feet. Hold the position for as long as possible.

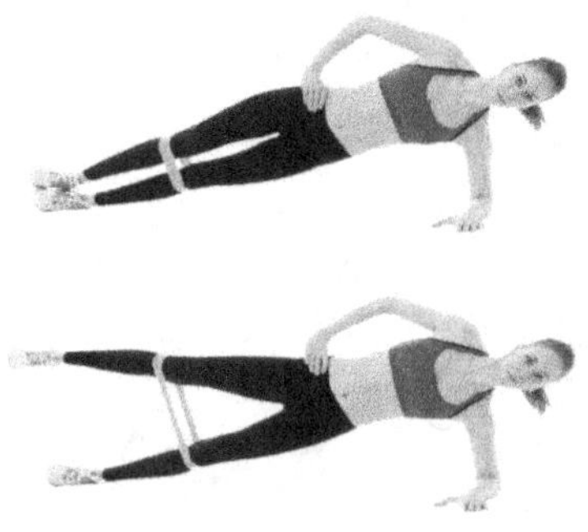

Crunch Exercises

Crunches

Lie on your back with your knees bent and your feet flat on the floor. Place a resistance band across the top of your back. Cross your arms across your chest or rest them behind your head. Engage your core and curl your upper body off the floor. Slowly decrease back down to the beginning position.

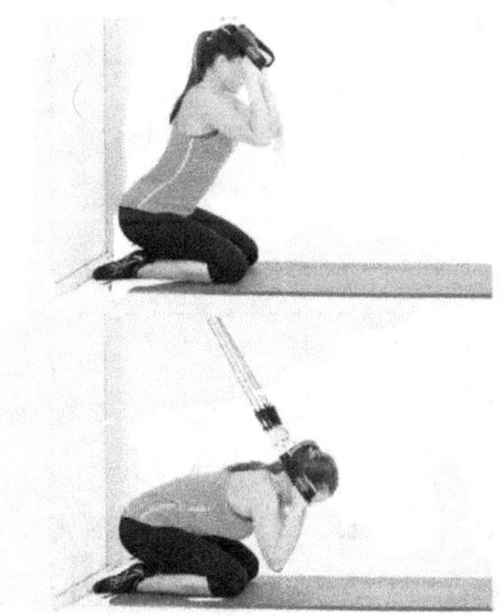

Reverse Crunches

Lie on your back with your legs outstretched and your feet flat on the floor. Place a resistance band around the soles of your feet. Engage your core and draw your knees towards your chest. Slowly lower your legs back to the starting position.

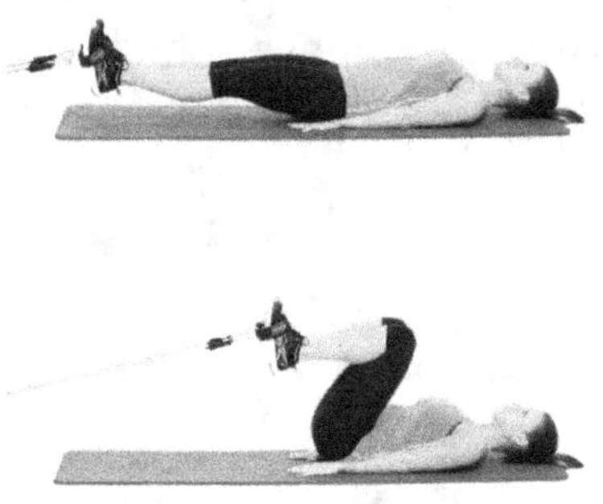

Bicycle Crunches

Lie on your back with your knees bent and your feet off the floor. Place your hands behind your head or cross them over your chest. Bring your right knee towards your chest while twisting your body to bring your left elbow closer to your right knee. Repeat on the opposite side.

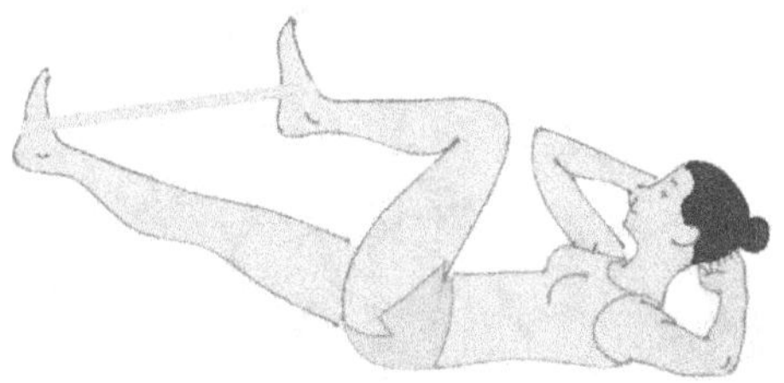

Russian Twists

Sit on the floor with your knees bent and your feet off the ground. Hold a resistance band in your hands and stretch your arms in front of you. Twist your body to the right, and then twist to the left.

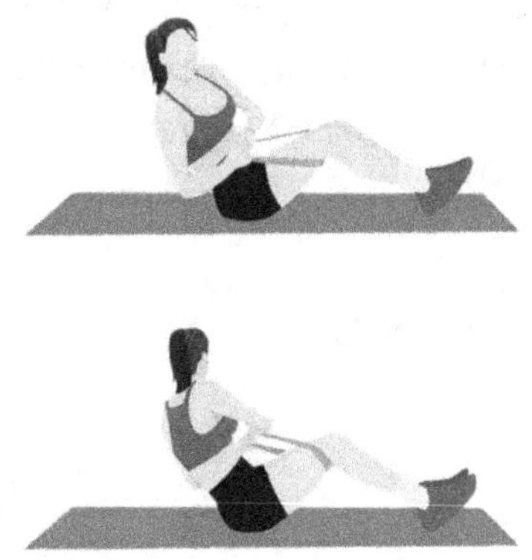

By adding these exercises into your training program, you may effectively target the main core muscles, boosting your stability, balance, and general fitness. Remember to maintain appropriate form during each exercise to minimize strain or injury.

Chapter 5: Workout Routines

With a variety of resistance band workouts available, choosing an effective training regimen is vital for accomplishing your fitness objectives. This chapter contains three example exercise routines customized to various fitness levels: beginner, moderate, and advanced.

Beginner Workout Routine

Frequency: 2-3 times each week

Warm-up: 5 minutes of easy exercise, such as walking or running in place

Workout:

Shoulder Press - 3 sets of 10-12 reps

Bicep Curls - 3 sets of 10-12 repetitions

Tricep Extensions - 3 sets of 10-12 repetitions

Squats - 3 sets of 10-12 repetitions

Lunges - 3 sets of 10-12 repetitions (per leg)

Calf Raises - 3 sets of 15-20 repetitions

Cool-down: 5 minutes of stretching

Intermediate Workout Routine

Frequency: 3-4 times per week

Warm-up: 5-10 minutes of easy exercise, such as jumping jacks or running in place

Workout:

Shoulder Press - 3 sets of 12-15 reps

Lateral Raises - 3 sets of 12-15 repetitions

Rear Delt Flyes - 3 sets of 12-15 repetitions

Bicep Curls - 3 sets of 12-15 repetitions

Tricep Extensions - 3 sets of 12-15 repetitions

Bent-Over Rows - 3 sets of 12-15 repetitions

Deadlifts - 3 sets of 10-12 repetitions

Leg Press - 3 sets of 12-15 repetitions

Glute Bridges - 3 sets of 15-20 repetitions

Calf Raises - 3 sets of 20-25 repetitions

Cool-down: 10 minutes of stretching

Advanced Workout Routine

Frequency: 3-5 times per week

Warm-up: 10-15 minutes of mild cardio, such as burpees or running in place

Workout:

Shoulder Press - 4 sets of 10-12 repetitions

Lateral Raises - 4 sets of 10-12 repetitions

Rear Delt Flyes - 4 sets of 10-12 repetitions

Bicep Curls - 4 sets of 10-12 repetitions

Tricep Extensions - 4 sets of 10-12 repetitions

Bent-Over Rows - 4 sets of 10-12 repetitions

Face Pulls - 3 sets of 15-20 repetitions

Deadlifts - 4 sets of 8-10 repetitions

Leg Extensions - 3 sets of 12-15 repetitions

Hamstring Curls - 3 sets of 12-15 repetitions

Hip Abduction - 3 sets of 12-15 reps (per leg)

Calf Raises - 3 sets of 25-30 repetitions

Cool-down: 15 minutes of vigorous stretching

These example training programs give a starting point for persons of all fitness levels. Remember to change the number of sets, repetitions, and resistance levels as required to fit your unique strength and endurance. Always listen to your body and rest when required to avoid overexertion or injury.

Chapter 6: Tips and Troubleshooting

Making the most of your resistance band exercises includes employing efficient tactics and overcoming frequent hurdles. This chapter gives important advice and troubleshooting solutions to improve your resistance band training experience.

Tips for Enhancing Resistance Band Workouts

Progressive Overload: Gradually increase the resistance, amount of repetitions, or sets over time to continually push your muscles and encourage strength growth.

Mind-Muscle Connection: Focus on activating the target muscle group throughout each exercise. This mind-muscle link boosts muscle activation and improves workout efficacy.

Controlled Tempo: Avoid jerky or hurried motions. Maintain a steady and smooth speed during each exercise to enhance muscle activation and reduce injury risk.

Good Form: Maintain good form and body alignment throughout each workout. This provides proper muscular activation and avoids strain or damage.

Breathing: Maintain steady breathing during each activity. Avoid holding your breath, since this might impede oxygen flow and impair workout performance.

Warm-up and Cool-down: Always include a warm-up before your exercise to prepare your muscles for action and a cool-down afterward to aid healing.

Range: Incorporate a range of resistance band workouts to target all main muscle groups and minimize boredom.

Rest and Recovery: enable appropriate rest and recovery between exercises to enable your muscles to heal and regenerate.

Troubleshooting Common Challenges

Resistance Band Selection: Choose the right resistance level depending on your fitness level. Starting with lighter bands and gradually increasing resistance minimizes overexertion and damage.

Band Placement: Position the resistance bands appropriately to achieve optimal muscle activation. Refer to workout descriptions or get help from a fitness expert.

Form Issues: If you encounter pain or discomfort during an activity, examine your form. Seek support from a fitness expert if required.

Plateaus: If you see a plateau in your development, try raising the resistance level, integrating new exercises, or increasing the number of sets or repetitions.

Motivation: Find techniques to retain motivation, such as establishing reasonable objectives, evaluating your progress, or finding an exercise partner.

Injuries: If you encounter any discomfort that lingers beyond the exercise, discontinue the activity and see a healthcare practitioner.

Remember, persistence and appropriate technique are crucial to reaching your fitness objectives with resistance band training. By following these guidelines and resolving frequent problems, you may enhance the efficacy and pleasure of your resistance band training session.

Conclusion

Embracing Consistency and Achieving Fitness Goals

Resistance band exercises provide a varied, effective, and accessible method to improve your physical well-being. To optimize the advantages of resistance band training, it is vital to embrace consistency, measure your progress, and establish reasonable objectives.

The Importance of Consistency

Consistency is the cornerstone of getting consistent fitness outcomes. By including resistance band exercises into your everyday routine, you offer your body with continual stimulation, resulting in incremental strength improvements, increased muscle tone, and enhanced overall fitness. Consistent training also helps develop exercise as an entrenched habit, fostering long-term commitment to a healthy lifestyle.

Tracking Your Progress

Monitoring your progress is vital for keeping motivation and analyzing the efficiency of your fitness plan. Keep a workout notebook to document the exercises you perform, the resistance levels you use, and the number of repetitions and sets completed. Tracking your progress helps you to discover areas for improvement and make modifications to your program as required.

Setting Realistic Goals

Setting realistic and attainable objectives gives guidance and inspiration throughout your fitness journey. Start with simple, reasonable objectives and progressively raise the difficulty as your strength and endurance develop. Celebrate your victories along the road to sustain motivation and reaffirm your dedication to your fitness ambitions.

Remember, resistance band exercises are a journey, not a destination. Embrace consistency, measure your progress, establish reasonable objectives, and enjoy the process of becoming a stronger, healthier version of yourself.

WEEKLY
Fitness Planner
Training Focus

Week Of:

Resistance Training

Exercise	Set	Rep	Weight

Strength Training

Exercise	Set	Rep	Duration

Notes

WEEKLY
Fitness Planner

Training Focus

Week Of :

Resistance Training

Exercise	Set	Rep	Weight

Strength Training

Exercise	Set	Rep	Duration

Notes

WEEKLY
Fitness Planner

Training Focus

Week Of :

Resistance Training

	Exercise	Set	Rep	Weight
☐				
☐				
☐				
☐				
☐				
☐				

Strength Training

	Exercise	Set	Rep	Duration
☐				
☐				
☐				
☐				
☐				
☐				

Notes

WEEKLY
Fitness Planner

Training Focus

Resistance Training

	Exercise	Set	Rep	Weight
☐				
☐				
☐				
☐				
☐				
☐				

Strength Training

	Exercise	Set	Rep	Duration
☐				
☐				
☐				
☐				
☐				
☐				

Notes

www.ingramcontent.com/pod-product-compliance
Lightning Source LLC
Chambersburg PA
CBHW070728260726
48660CB00007B/2767